OZONE, UV AND YOUR HEALTH

50 WAYS TO SAVE YOUR SKIN

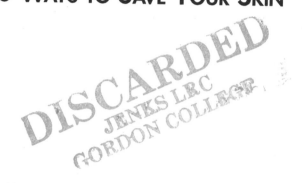
BY BUCK TILTON AND ROGER G. COX

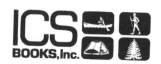

ICS BOOKS, Inc.
Merrillville, Indiana

DEDICATION

We dedicate this book to our families,
and to all the families of the world.
We live under the same bright sun.

recycled paper

All ICS titles are printed on 50% recycled paper from pre-
consumer waste. All sheets are processed without using acid.

PUBLISHED BY:
ICS Books, Inc.
1370 E. 86th Place
Merrillville, IN 46410
800-541-7323

Library of Congress Cataloging-in-Publication Data
Tilton, Buck.
       Ozone, UV and your health : 50 ways to save your skin /
    Buck Tilton and Roger G. Cox.
          p. cm.
       Includes index.
       ISBN: 0-934802-95-5
       1. Ultraviolet radiation—Health aspects. 2. Ozone layer depletion—
Health aspects. I. Cox, Roger. 1947– . II. Title.
QP82.2.U4T55 1994
616.5—dc20   93-49775
                                                      CIP

TABLE OF CONTENTS

UV and your Eyes

UV and Your Lifestyle

INTRODUCTION

HOW UV AND OZONE AFFECT YOUR HEALTH

While recent dramatic rises in skin cancer rates are primarily due to an increase in outdoor recreational lifestyles, scientists and doctors are now concerned about a new cause of increased ultraviolet (UV) radiation exposure—the thinning of Earth's natural protective ozone shield. To help you better understand the health hazards from the UV and ozone connection, let's quickly review some science and history.

Compared to quantities of other gases (oxygen, nitrogen, and carbon dioxide), ozone molecules are quite rare in our atmosphere—but they provide a critical protective function for most lifeforms on our planet. Most of the Earth's ozone (about 90 percent) resides in the stratosphere, located 6 to 25 miles above the Earth's surface. Ozone's unique optical properties allow it to serve as a shield from dangerous UV radiation. An ozone molecule consists of three oxygen atoms. The so called "stratospheric ozone shield" is a thin layer of ozone molecules. The stratospheric ozone layer is actually very thin—if all the ozone molecules over your head were compressed together with sea-level pressure, they would form a layer less than 1/8 inch (3 millimeters) thick.

Solar radiation—a fancy word for sunlight—is made up of rays with many different wavelengths. Some you can see with your eyes, some are invisible. Wavelengths are measured in nanometers (nm). Here is how different wavelengths compare:

Above 700 nm	Infrared (invisible heat rays)
650 to 700 nm	Red light
590 to 650 nm	Orange light
490 to 590 nm	Yellow and Green light
420 to 490 nm	Blue light
400 to 420 nm	Violet light
Below 400 nm	Ultraviolet (invisible UV rays)

The sun's rays are essential for both plant and animal life, but the very short UV wavelengths can actually damage living cells. The ozone layer allows life to flourish on Earth by passing the longer, beneficial wavelengths and effectively blocking the shorter UV waves. The shortest UV wavelengths are the most damaging—they contain enough energy to actually destroy DNA molecules in your skin and eyes. Since DNA controls your cells' ability to heal and reproduce, it's no wonder that overexposure to UV rays is dangerous.

Ultraviolet rays are divided into three groups by scientists according to their wavelength and relative hazard to your health. None are visible to the human eye:

320 to 400 nm	UVA: Beneficial in low doses, may cause cancer
280 to 320 nm	UVB: Causes sunburns and cancer
below 280 nm	UVC: Quickly causes burns and cancers

Almost all UVA radiation passes through the ozone shield and, as far as science is concerned, it always has. Ozone effectively blocks nearly all UVC. It also does a good job of protecting us from excessive UVB radiation—if the shield is undamaged and can do its job. Unfortunately, in the last 10 years the ozone layer has started to thin as manmade CFC chemicals attack the ozone.

A QUICK HISTORY: CFCs AND THE OZONE SHIELD

Ozone is blue gas with a pungent odor. It gets its name from a Greek word meaning "smell." The gas was discovered in the 1840s, and by the early 1880s, scientists had already identified the stratospheric ozone shield, and understood its ability to block UV radiation.

Ozone is formed in the upper atmosphere by the action of sunlight on ordinary oxygen molecules. Sunlight splits apart oxygen molecules into single oxygen atoms. These atoms then bond to nearby oxygen molecules creating the three-atom ozone molecule. While this mechanism creates new ozone molecules, chemical reactions with naturally occurring compounds are constantly destroying ozone. Normally, the delicate balance in the thickness of the ozone shield is maintained with only minor fluctuations due to sunspots or volcanic activity.

Manmade chemicals are seldom found in the stratosphere because of the intense levels of UV radiation. High-energy UV sunlight breaks down most compounds into elemental atoms at much lower altitudes. Unfortunately, one class of manmade chemicals, halocarbons, are so stable that they do not break down until they reach the stratosphere. The best known types of halocarbons are chlorofluorocarbons (CFCs) used for refrigeration, air conditioning, plastic foams, and as industrial cleaners. Halocarbons contain either chlorine or bromine. Other halocarbons include halons, carbon tetrachloride, and methyl chloroform. CFCs were invented by the DuPont Corporation in the 1930s for use in refrigeration. DuPont sold the chemicals under the trademarked name Freon. At that time they appeared to be "ideal chemicals", because CFCs are non-toxic and non-combustible.

In 1974, two chemists, Sherry Rowland and Mario Molina, working at the University of California at Irvine, determined that CFCs could be a potential threat to the ozone layer. They showed that if CFCs released their chlorine atoms in the stratosphere, this extra chlorine could become a catalyst to greatly accelerate ozone destruction. The chemists produced in their laboratory the ozone-destroying reactions they feared were occurring in the upper atmosphere, but their warnings were ignored by the chemical industry and government. As a result CFC production continued to grow.

By 1985, a British team of scientists made public their measurements that showed a significant drop in ozone levels at their Antarctic research station at Halley Bay. The reductions were very dramatic during the month of October, which is springtime in Antarctica. Soon NASA's Nimbus series of satellites confirmed the ozone loss, and full-color images of Antarctic ozone holes were generated. Now scientists needed to determine if the ozone loss was due to CFCs as Roland and Molina suspected. In August and September of 1987, NASA used high-altitude aircraft to fly through the hole while scientists measured levels of chlorine and ozone. Direct atmospheric measurements proved manmade CFCs were the culprit.

Since that discovery, governments around the world have scrambled to slow and eventually stop the production of CFCs and halons. The Montreal Protocol in 1988 was the first step, calling for reduced CFC production. But each year since 1985 ozone levels worldwide have continued to drop, and the Protocol has been revised with the London (1990) and Copenhagen (1992) Amendments. Under the Copenhagen Amendment, most CFCs will be phased out by 1996, but other chlorine compounds will not be phased out until the year 2015, and some chemicals are still not regulated at all.

WHAT TO EXPECT IN THE FUTURE

The South Pole ozone hole was discovered unexpectedly in the early 1980s, and scientists still do not fully understand what will happen to the ozone layer in the future. However, a number of basic facts are known: 1) The CFC chemicals causing the ozone destruction are still accumulating in the stratosphere and CFC levels will not begin to fall for at least 10 more years. 2) When CFC levels begin to fall, they will fall slowly, and it will take until the year 2060 before they reach the levels of the early 1980s. 3) Antarctic ozone holes become larger each year, last longer, and are becoming more severe. 4) Ozone levels are decreasing on a worldwide basis. 5) As ozone levels decrease, measured UVB levels are increasing, and can be expected to increase for at least 15 to 20 more years.

The situation is not encouraging. The CFC "genie" has been let out of the bottle, and despite the recent attempts to stop CFC production, we will all have to cope with increased levels of UVB radiation in the future. Since ozone levels fluctuate in seasonal patterns, depend on latitude, and drop rapidly during ozone hole episodes, governments have begun to include UV radiation forecasts as a standard part of daily local weather forecasts. Canada and Australia already do this, and in the United States, the National Weather Service and the National Oceanic and Atmospheric Administration (NOAA) will probably begin a similar UV advisory program in 1994. The program will use the same UV Index system being used now by Canada.

The purpose of this book is to help you protect yourself and your family from the damaging effects of UV radiation. One way to do this is to understand the UV Index numbers and forecasts, and know how to minimize your UV exposure risks.

RESOURCES

Carl Zimmer, "Son of Ozone Hole," *Discover* (October 1993): 27-28.

J.F. Gleason, et al., "Record Low Global Ozone in 1992," *Science* 260 (April 23, 1993): 523-526.

Thomas Kamm, "Sheep and Trees Are Acting Strangely After a Hole Opens in Ozone at 'End of the World' in South Chile," *Wall Street Journal* (January 12, 1993): 1,8.

J. D. Mahlman, "A Looming Arctic Ozone Hole," *Nature* 360 (November 19, 1992): 209.

Susan Solomon & Daniel L.. Albritton, "Time-Dependent Ozone Depletion Potentials for Short- and Long-term Forecasts," *Nature* 357 (May 7, 1992): 33-37.

Richard Stolarski et. al., "Measured Trends in Stratospheric Ozone," *Science* 256 (April 17, 1992): 342-349.

UV, You and The UV Index

1 Understand UV Index Forecasts

The UV Index is a method for measuring the strength of UVB radiation on any given day. The UV Index is a scale that usually runs from 1 to 10, but Index values as high as 11 or 12 are possible in tropical regions. The UV Index number is given as a daily forecast, or for a reading of the previous day. The number represents the highest UVB level reached for the day, which will occur at solar noon (see 2. Solar Noon) under clear skies.

As mentioned in the Introduction, the UV Index system was first used in Canada, and is now being introduced into the United States. In the U.S., the UV Index data is generated by the National Weather Service and National Oceanic Atmospheric Administration (NOAA) using real-time ozone data collected from NOAA satellites.

You may also be aware of UV readings broadcast on your local TV station that use the Sunsor scale. Sunsor is a registered trademark of the Sunsor Corporation, a private company that produces UV measuring equipment and works with many local TV stations to provide UVB intensity information. The Sunsor system uses a proprietary scale of 0 to 120, but the purpose is the same as the UV Index—to give you an idea of how strong the sun's UVB rays are. Since both systems are measuring the burning-type UVB radiation, Sunsor readings are roughly (but probably not exactly) ten times an equivalent UV Index reading.

RESOURCES

National Weather Service/NOAA, Climate Analysis, 5200 Auth Road, Room 805, Washington, DC 20233. (301) 763-8071

Sunsor, Inc., 1388 Freeport Road, Pittsburgh, PA 15238.

2 SOLAR NOON

"Do you remember how the sheriff (Gary Cooper) couldn't get anyone to come outside and help him fight the bad guys in the movie High Noon?"

–Paul G. Gill, Jr., M.D.

The sun's rays are strongest when the sun is highest in the sky. This occurs at midday, a time known as "solar noon." You will sunburn most easily at midday, so be sure to be well protected, if you must be outside at this time. On days when the UV Index is high, it is better to remain indoors or in deep shade during this period.

The UV Index numbers are given for solar noon each day. They represent the maximum UV intensity level forecast for that day.

WHAT TO DO

Solar noon does not usually occur at exactly 12:00 local time. It varies with your location, the time of year, and whether your location uses daylight savings time. For example, on June 21 in Altanta, solar noon occurs at 1:38PM local time. One way to estimate solar noon at your location is to look at the daily sunrise and sunset times in your local newspaper, then calculate the time exactly halfway between sunrise and sunset. This is when solar noon occurs and UV rays are the strongest.

RESOURCES

Computer programs are available for calculating the time of solar noon for different locations, along with other useful solar information:

UV B-WARE™: Save the Planet Software, P.O. Box 45, Pitkin, CO 81241. (303) 641-5035.

ASTROCALC: Zephyr Services, 1900 Murray Avenue, Pittsburgh, PA 15217.

3 UV LEVELS AND SUNBURN TIMES

"With a microwave oven, cooking times are measured in minutes. When UV radiation levels are high, your sunburn time is just minutes, too."

– Anonymous sunbather

If you know what the UV Index level is, you can estimate your sunburn time using the chart below. These sunburn times attempt to estimate when the first noticeable reddening occurs on Type III (see 13. Type Is Only Skin Deep) untanned Caucasian skin. They were derived from approximate guidelines used by both the Australian and Canadian governments to explain UV Index levels. Keep in mind that more sensitive skin types will burn in a shorter time, while people with darker skin can tolerate longer exposures.

UV INDEX	SUNBURN TIME
10	13 minutes
8	17 minutes
6	22 minutes
4	34 minutes
2	67 minutes

RESOURCE

Atmospheric Environment Service, Environment Canada, 4905 Dufferin St., Downsview, Ontario M3H 5T4.

4 CLOUDS AND UV LEVELS

Clouds provide some shade, but very little UV protection. You are probably well aware that you can get sunburned on a cloudy day because most clouds do a poor job of blocking UVB rays. In fact, on a bright day with fluffy cumulus clouds in the sky, you can actually receive an increased dose of UVB—as much as 15% more. This is because scattered UV is reflected down to earth by these white clouds. Only thick, dark rain clouds offer much UV protection—and these are the days when you are probably covered up with a windbreaker or rain jacket anyway.

You can sunburn your skin easily on cloudy summer days because the clouds make the air cooler by blocking heat-carrying infrared rays, and you are usually not as aware of the burning effect of the sun's rays on your skin

WHAT TO DO

Don't ever rely on cloud cover to protect your skin and eyes. Always use a hat, sunscreen and sunglasses—unless you are walking in the rain with your raincoat or umbrella.

RESOURCE

"Solar power," by Paul Gill, Jr., M.D. *Outdoor Life,* June 1993.

5 CHANGING SEASONS AND UV LEVELS

UV levels depend on both the seasonal strength of the sun and the seasonal thickness of the ozone shield. Although the sun is closer to the earth in winter, it is more directly overhead in summer. Summertime in North America brings more sunshine, warmer weather, and the highest UV levels of the year. Although the longest day of the year occurs at the summer solstice—usually June 21—the maximum UV levels do not peak in most U.S. cities until sometime in mid-July. The reason for this is the seasonal fluctuation of ozone levels. Ozone levels are highest in early spring, then drop during the summer, reaching their lowest levels in November or December.

The range of UV fluctuation from summer to winter depends on the latitude of your location. For example, the UV index in San Francisco typically peaks around 8.8 in July and drops to just below 2 in December and January. In Tampa, Florida, the index hits a high of 10 in July, stays above 9 for twelve weeks, and drops to about 4 in December.

WHAT TO DO

Scientists studying the ozone depletion problem have measured reduction in ozone values during all seasons, but the biggest reductions have occurred in the spring months for the U.S. and Canada. Be especially careful about sun exposure anytime from early March through October.

RESOURCE

National Weather Service/NOAA, Climate Analysis, 5200 Auth Road, Room 805, Washington, DC 20233. (301) 763-8071.

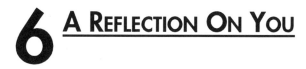

6 A REFLECTION ON YOU

Exposure to ultraviolet radiation can be increased by reflection of the damaging rays from natural and man-made surfaces. Bright metal and white-painted surfaces can reflect a significant amount of UV radiation. Grass reflects from 2.5-3%, sand 20-30%, snow and ice from 80-90%. Depending on the angle of reflection, water can reflect up to 100% of the UV rays striking its surface. The angle of reflection is determined in part by the height of the sun above the horizon. Early in the morning and late in the evening, with the sun low in the sky, water may reflect only 10% of the UV rays. At noon, with the sun directly overhead and striking vertically, water absorbs most of the UV light, and reflection may drop to 5%. Mid-morning and mid-afternoon, with the sun at a 35-45 degree angle, water's reflection is at its greatest. If the water is choppy, the reflective surface increases, and reflection is even higher than when water is calm.

Reflection of UV rays is maximized when you're traveling in a snow-filled bowl high in the mountains. More UV radiation reaches the ground at higher altitudes. Much of the UV radiation is reflected by the snow. The rounded terrain focuses much of the reflected UV light on you.

WHAT TO DO

Remember that shade may not be as protective as you think. Protect your skin with sunscreens and clothing, your eyes with sunglasses, if you are working or playing on or near reflective surfaces. Don't forget the bottom of your nose and chin where reflected UV radiation can burn you.

RESOURCES

Management of Wilderness and Environmental Emergencies, edited by Paul Auerbach, MD, and Edward Geehr, MD. The C. V. Mosby Company, 11830 Westline Industrial Drive, St. Louis, MO 63146.

"Wilderness Eye Protection," by Stephen R. Chun, O.D. *Wilderness First Aid,* P. O. Box 1227, Berkeley, CA 94701. Spring 1990 issue.

7 ALTITUDE AND UV LEVELS

"The higher you are, the closer the sun."

– Mary Roach

While most ozone is located in the stratosphere, some ozone occurs in the air at all altitudes. UV rays are filtered out by the total amount of ozone from ground level up to the upper stratosphere. Scientists call this the "total ozone column." At higher elevations there is less total atmosphere above your head, so the total ozone column reading is lower, allowing more UV radiation to reach you.

Researchers from Canada's Atmospheric Service estimate that UV levels increase about 7% for each 3,300 feet (1 km) of altitude. Some experts say there can be as much as 4 to 5% increase for every 1000 feet of elevation gain. This means when you are skiing in the Colorado or Utah mountains you are getting at least 20 to 25% more UV exposure than you would at sea-level for a similar latitude location.

WHAT TO DO

Take special precautions when skiing, hiking, or climbing in the mountains. Be sure your sunglasses or goggles offer side protection. Use a hat and be sure to cover your neck. Remember that in addition to the higher risks of UV directly due to altitude, you also face additional exposure due to reflected sunlight off of snow and ice.

RESOURCES

Atmosphere Environmental Service, Environment Canada, 4905 Dufferin Street, Downsview, Ontario M3H 5T4.

"Sun Struck," by Mary Roach, *Health,* May/June 1992.

8 CHANGES IN LATITUDE, CHANGES IN UV ATTITUDE

Jimmy Buffet and your fifth-grade geography teacher were both right—there is more sunshine in Mexico than in Chicago. Locations close to the equator receive the most annual sunshine, while areas close to the poles receive relatively small amounts of solar radiation. This is due to the angle of the sun varying with latitude. In polar areas the sun is always low on the horizon, while at the equator, the sun is high in the sky every day, and it shines intensely.

Stronger sunlight means higher levels of cancer-causing UVB radiation. The annual UVB dosage level in Dallas is approximately 38% higher than in Boston. Stronger UV rays translate directly to more cases of skin cancer. There have been 47% more cases of skin cancer reported in Dallas than in Boston. Researchers from the U.S. Department of Health, Education, and Welfare (HEW), Public Health Service, and National Institutes of Health (NIH) tabulated the skin cancer rates for white males on a state-by-state basis. Then they plotted the cancer rates for each state according to the latitude for each individual state. Cancer rates in the southern states of Texas and Florida are approximately twice as high as the rates for the northern states of Wisconsin and Montana. The connection between high UVB and high cancer rates is well documented.

WHAT TO DO

As you travel south, stay aware of higher UV levels associated with these lower latitudes. It's easier to get a bad sunburn in these warmer regions—even during the winter months.

RESOURCE

Biological Effects of Ultraviolet Radiation, by Walter Harm. Cambridge University Press, 32 East 57th Street, New York, NY 10022.

9 BURNING IN THE WIND

Wind, all by itself, does not cause your skin to burn, although it can cause drying and chapping. But wind and UV radiation at the same time work together to make your sunburn worse. A term for the ill effects of wind and sun is "windburn." The combination of wind and sun can be harmful due to:

1) The acceleration of the drying of sweat from your skin, which removes urocanic acid, a naturally-occurring chemical in your skin that helps protect you from UV radiation.

2) The feeling of coolness that wind produces, causing you to expose your skin to the sun longer than you otherwise would.

3) The irritative effect of wind on skin that intensifies sunburn.

RESOURCE

The Waterlover's Guide to Marine Medicine, by Paul Gill, Jr., M.D. Simon & Schuster, Rockefeller Center, 1230 Avenue of the Americas, New York, NY 10020.

10 MID-DAY UV EXPOSURE

When is the best time to be indoors or in deep shade? Many experts say you should try to avoid direct sun exposure between the hours of 10AM and 3PM. Another rule-of-thumb is to avoid being outdoors for the two hours before solar noon and the two hours after solar noon. At other hours of the day, the sun may be only 70% as strong as its highest intensity at solar noon. If you avoid exposure for 3 hours before, and 3 hours after solar noon, you will only be exposed to UV levels less than half as intense as mid-day levels.

WHAT TO DO

Since it's easier to get sunburned in the middle of the day, you can reduce your UV exposure risks by scheduling some of your regular outdoor activities in the morning or late afternoon. This is especially true in the late spring and during the summer months when mid-day UV levels are very high. For example, if your summer exercise routine includes a jog or bike ride, you could greatly reduce your UV dosage and health risks by shifting these activities from your lunch hour to a time before or after work.

When hiking or backpacking in the spring and summer months, take a long lunch break (or a short nap) in a shady spot, to avoid the heat and high UV radiation of the noontime sun.

11 URBAN POLLUTION IS NOT THE SOLUTION

While most ozone resides in the stratospheric ozone layer miles above our heads, there is also ozone located near ground level. The low-level ozone is called tropospheric ozone. Most tropospheric ozone is created by industrial pollution and automobile exhaust gases. Tropospheric ozone levels are much higher in large, congested urban cities than in urban areas.

Measurements in some large cities show the additional ozone created at ground level has partially compensated for the thinning of the stratospheric ozone layer, resulting in only small increases in UV levels. That sounds like good news—a manmade ozone shield—but, unfortunately, this is not the case. Ozone is a nasty pollutant when it occurs at ground level. Exposure to ozone causes eye irritation, lung damage and other health problems.

WHAT TO DO

Don't rely on urban air pollution to save your skin from UV rays—you will be subjecting yourself to additional health risks in heavily polluted, high-traffic urban areas. When vacationing in rural and wilderness areas, remember to protect your skin with proper clothing and sunscreen—the sun's UV rays are stronger without the blanket of urban smog.

12 LOOK THROUGH ANY WINDOW

Glass in the windows of your house blocks UVB radiation, the kind most suspect in sunburn and cancer. If you enjoy sitting in the sun, at ease in your favorite chair, with warm sunshine beaming across your shoulder, keep it up. There is very little chance of skin damage.

Glass protects you from UV radiation better than plastic, in general, but most plastics are treated with UV absorbers so they will last longer. Safety glass in car windows has a layer of plastic built in to keep the glass from shattering on impact. Car interiors are relatively free of UV light . . . unless you're riding in a convertible with the top down.

RESOURCE

"Sun Struck," by Mary Roach. *Health,* May/June 1992.

UV AND YOUR SKIN

13 TYPE IS ONLY SKIN DEEP

Not all skins are created equal. The more sensitive your skin, the more careful you need to be. Naturally dark-skinned people have high concentrations of melanin in their skin, which absorbs UV radiation, so they suffer less from sunburn, skin cancer, and sun-induced aging with its subsequent wrinkling.

TYPE	CHARACTERISTICS	EXAMPLES
I	Burns easily, never tans	Blondes, red heads, blue-eyed
II	Burns usually, tans after long hours of exposure	Fair skinned, blondes
III	Burns and tans moderately	Most Caucasians
IV	Burns a little, tans well	Hispanics, Asians
V	Burns rarely, tans darkly	Middle Easterners, Indians
VI	Burns only after extreme exposure	Blacks

RESOURCE

Paul G. Gill, Jr., M.D., author of *Pocket Guide to Wilderness Medicine,* available from Dr. Gill, Box 56, Middlebury, VT 05753. $11.95 postpaid.

14 SUNBURN

"Alas, the sun is about as healthy as smoking cigarettes."
–Karl Neumann, M.D.

Ultraviolet radiation from the sun, striking human skin, is partly reflected, partly absorbed by outer layers, and partly transmitted to deeper layers until its energy dissipates. UV rays will traumatize your skin when exposure time is long enough, and the result is called "sunburn." Ultraviolet B (UVB) rays are the primary skin burners, but UVA can augment the power of UVB. Mild redness of the skin can occur in a brief period of exposure, but true sunburn takes more time. The amount of time it takes to burn skin varies greatly, but most white-skinned people will experience some true sunburn in approximately 20 minutes of exposure of a previously unexposed area (say the buttock) to mid-summer mid-day sun. Black-skinned people may take 30 times longer to burn.

True sunburn begins to appear 2-8 hours after exposure, and reaches maximum intensity somewhere between 24 and 36 hours after exposure. Evidence of damage to the epidermis, the outer skin, is predominantly cellular and persists for 3-7 days. Damage to the dermis, the true skin, is predominantly vascular and persists for 3-5 days.

WHAT TO DO

Sunburn produces first or second degree damage to skin: painful redness, swelling, blisters, skin peeling. If you are sunburned, take aspirin or ibuprofen (e.g. Advil) for pain and itching. The recommended doses are: about 650 mgs aspirin or about 400 mgs ibuprofen every four hours for 24 hours. For severe itching, take an antihistamine, such as diphenhydramine (e.g. Benadryl). Do not take any medication if you are allergic to it. Creams and ointments, available over-the-counter, that contain cortisone give the most effective relief. Stronger medications are available from your doctor. Baths or compresses of cool or lukewarm water often provide some relief. While your damaged skin heals, application of other substances—topical anesthetics, perfume, insect repellents, calamine lotion, even sunscreens—may be dangerous, since your skin has increased sensitivity and increased ability to absorb substances. Severe sunburn, involving oozing blisters, should be seen promptly by a physician.

There is nothing healthy about burned skin. Although sunburn is transient short-term skin damage, long-term effects may show up later, including premature skin aging and skin cancer. Avoid sunburn.

RESOURCES

Management of Wilderness and Environmental Emergencies, edited by Paul Auerbach, M.D., and Edward Geehr, M.D. The C. V. Mosby Company, 11830 Westline Industrial Drive, St. Louis, MO 63146.

Traveling Healthy, Volume 2, Number 3, edited by Karl Neumann, M.D. 108-48 70th Road, Forest Hills, NY 11375.

15 AGE BEFORE BEAUTY

"Not only can excessive solar exposure accelerate and intensify aging in skin, it can also lead to serious health risks."

–John Browder, M.D. and Betsy Beers, M.D.

Somewhere between the transient pain and redness of sunburn and the malignant cancer of melanoma lies photoaging, the changes that occur in human skin with cumulative exposure to solar light. UV light, absorbed by your skin, leads to permanent damage to RNA and DNA, alterations in connective tissue, and loss of stabilization in membranes. These changes may make little or no difference in the way you function, but they can profoundly change the way you look.

Intrinsic skin changes are just a part of the natural aging process, but they are accelerated in photodamaged skin. Extrinsic skin changes are caused by exposure to things in your environment: heat, wind, some chemicals, cigarette smoke and, by far the most significant, UV radiation. These changes include fine and deep wrinkling, pigment alterations (including permanent spots and the red leathery skin of cutis rhomboidalis from which we get the term "redneck"), sagging, and changes in the vasculature of the skin. Elastosis, increased numbers of altered elastic fibers, is the most universal sign of photoaging. You don't see elastosis in unexposed areas of your body.

WHAT TO DO

To stop photoaging, you must stop exposing your unprotected skin to solar radiation. Use sunscreens and protective clothing, and avoid the mid-day sun. Although most photoaging is permanent, some changes are reversible with cessation of exposure.

RESOURCES

"Photoaging" by John Browder, M.D. and Betsy Beers, M.D. *Postgraduate Medicine,* Volume 93, Number 8.

16 BASAL CELL CARCINOMA

"By far the most common cause of skin cancer is overexposure to the sun."

– American Cancer Society

Skin cancer is the most common form of cancer, with over 600,000 new cases reported every year. It's the fastest growing form of cancer, 14 times more common than 60 years ago. Fortunately, it's one of the most curable forms of cancer, if detected early enough. It is also preventable.

Of the three major types of skin cancer, basal cell cancer ranks as the one most commonly diagnosed. About one half million cases are reported annually. Your basal cells make up the base of your epidermis. If too much UV radiation causes those cells to reproduce too fast (while at the same time repressing your natural immune response to such unnatural reproduction), a tumorous growth forms. Basal cell carcinoma usually start as a slow-growing, small, shiny (or pearly) bump or nodule that becomes an open sore taking longer than three weeks to heal. They often bleed, crust over, and open to bleed again. The cancer may be an itchy or tender reddish patch that comes and goes. Sometimes it's a pale splotch, like a scar, and sometimes a circular growth with a raised border and depressed center.

On rare occasions, these cancerous basal cells release from the tumor, usually into your blood, and take up residence in another organ, such as your liver. The cancer is said to have metastasized, and it is now a threat to your life. The survival rate of treated basal cell carcinoma, before it has a chance to metastasize, is greater than 95%. Unfortunately, the problem shows up again in one out of every three to five survivors.

WHAT TO DO

If you suspect you have skin cancer, see your doctor as soon as possible. In the meantime, do not overexpose your unprotected skin to ultraviolet rays.

RESOURCES

American Cancer Society. (800) 227-2345.

"Basal Cell Carcinoma," by Steven Hacker, MD, John Browder, MD, Francisco Ramos-Caro, MD. *Postgraduate Medicine,* Volume 93, Number 8, June 1993.

National Cancer Institute. (800) 422-6237.

17 SQUAMOUS CELL CARCINOMA

"Ninety percent of all skin cancers occur on parts of the body that usually aren't covered by clothing."
– American Cancer Society

Usual sites for skin cancer are the face, ears, hands and forearms. In the past 50 years, shoulders, backs and chests on men, and the lower legs on women, have become increasingly common sites for skin cancer. The reason, of course: deliberate exposure of those body parts to the sun's ultraviolet radiation.

Of the three major types of skin cancer, squamous cell cancer ranks as the second most common, accounting for about 100,000 cases every year. Although not as common as basal cell carcinoma, its rate of increase is higher. Your squamous cells make up most of your epidermis, and they are susceptible to the same UV alterations as basal cells. This cancer may look like basal cell cancer, but it can also appear as a wart that bleeds and crusts over, bleeds and crusts over.

Cancerous squamous cells grow faster and metastasize more frequently than basal cell carcinoma, and over 2000 people will die from the problem this year. Still, the survival rate of treated squamous cell carcinoma, before it has a chance to metastasize, is greater than 90%. Unfortunately, this cancer shows up again at about the same rate as basal cell carcinoma.

WHAT TO DO

If you suspect you have skin cancer, see your doctor as soon as possible. In the meantime, do not overexpose your unprotected skin to ultraviolet rays. Squamous cell carcinoma may also result from overexposure to x-rays and certain chemical compounds such as coal tar, asphalt and pitch.

RESOURCES

American Cancer Society. (800) 227-2345.

National Cancer Institute. (800) 422-6237.

"Squamous Cell Carcinoma of the Skin," by Steven Hacker, M.D., and Franklin Flowers, M.D. *Postgraduate Medicine,* Volume 93, Number 8, June 1993.

18 MALIGNANT MELANOMA

"By the year 2000, projections suggest that malignant melanoma will affect 1 of every 90 Americans."
— Franklin S. Glickman, M.D.

Physicians employ several different techniques to remove skin cancer. The choice depends on the extent of the cancer, the position on the body, and the risks to the patient. Surgical removal accounts for 95% of treatments. Electrosurgery may be used, in which an electric current burns the border of the removal site to kill any remaining cancer. For those people who can't tolerate regular surgery, the cancer may be frozen and removed via a technique called cryosurgery. Another option, used most often in elderly patients, is radiation therapy, in which a beam of radiation, directed at the cancer, kills the bad cells. After it has metastasized, a melanoma usually requires chemotherapy or immunotherapy.

Of the three major types of skin cancer, malignant melanoma is the least common and the most serious. About 30,000 new cases appear each year. Melanomas involve your melanocytes, the cells that give your skin its color. This cancer most often originates in or near a mole, birthmark or "beauty mark." The more moles you have, the greater your risk of melanoma. But it can also occur as a new spot, and range in color from black to brown to red and blue to translucent. After they appear, they continue to grow with irregular borders.

Malignant melanoma kills nearly 7000 people every year. One in five diagnosed with malignant melanoma are dead within five years. But detected early, this cancer is cured almost 100% of the time. There is about a 50/50 chance of recurrence. Instead of cumulative exposure, malignant melanoma appears more often in people who have a history of serious sunburns, especially when they were children. If someone in your family has had this cancer, your risks are even higher. Women get it more often than men, especially women who have been on birth control pills for several years, and women who have given birth after the age of 30.

WHAT TO DO

The American Cancer Society recommends regularly checking yourself for The ABCDs of Early Detection.

A for Asymmetry: one half of the growth doesn't look like the other half.

B for Border: edges are ragged, irregular or indistinct.

C for Color: non-uniform pigmentation.

D for Diameter: any growth larger than 1/4 inch (6mm) should be checked.

RESOURCES

American Cancer Society. (800) 227-2345.

"Malignant Melanoma," by Franklin S. Glickman, M.D. *Family Practice Recertification,* Volume 15, Number 9, September 1993.

Skin Cancer Foundation, Box 561, New York, NY 10156.

19 SOLAR KERATOSES

"Regular use of sunscreens prevents the development of solar keratoses and, by implication, possibly reduces the risk of skin cancer in the long term."

— Thompson, et al.

Solar, or actinic, keratoses are horny growths that develop on human skin (most often the face, neck and back of the hands) from overexposure to ultraviolet light. They are becoming so common some doctors suggest 50% of all white-skinned people over the age of 40 have them, or will have them. Solar keratoses are pre-cancerous, non-malignant thickenings, but they are a powerful warning sign that skin cancer may be on the way.

Solar keratoses can be prevented in a large number of people with the regular use of sunscreens. People who already have solar keratoses sometimes see remission with the use of sunscreens. Although sunscreens are rated on their ability to prevent sunburn, not keratoses or cancer, studies show that higher SPFs do prevent keratoses in many people, and it is relatively safe to assume screens help prevent skin cancer as well.

WHAT TO DO

1. Use a sunscreen with a high SPF (at least 15) that protects against UVA and UVB every day you're exposed to ultraviolet light.

2. If you develop what you think are solar keratoses, see your doctor for an evaluation. They should be treated before they have a chance to degenerate into cancer.

RESOURCES

"Reduction of Solar Keratoses by Regular Sunscreen Use." by Sandra Thompson, Damien Jolley and Robin Marks. *New England Journal of Medicine,* Volume 329, Number 16, 14 October 1993.

The Waterlover's Guide to Marine Medicine, by Paul Gill, Jr., M.D. Simon & Schuster, Rockefeller Center, 1230 Avenue of the Americas, New York, NY 10020.

20 PHOTOSENSITIVITY

If you're taking a drug for a medical condition, using certain chemicals on your skin, or eating certain foods, you may be more than normally sensitive to the sun's ultraviolet radiation, or photosensitive. Problems of photosensitivity do not fall neatly into scientific classifications due to a wide variety of individual responses and lack of medical knowledge on the subject. But, generally, photosensitivity reactions fall into three broad categories: 1) Phototoxic reactions, an exaggerated normal response to sunlight, a common result of using some shampoos, perfumes and other everyday products. 2) Photoallergic reactions, an abnormal response to sunlight, usually a rash, from many medications, soaps and cosmetics. And 3) Phytophotodermatitis, a reaction from getting some plant juices on your skin prior to exposure to UV light, commonly caused by lemons, limes, celery, parsley, parsnips, carrots, figs and mustard.

A Partial List of Substances that May Cause Photosensitivity

Food additives, including cyclamates and saccharine.

Benzocaine, used in most anesthetic sprays.

Biothionol, used in some soaps and first aid creams.

Green soap.

Sunscreens, especially the ones with PABA.

A Partial List of Drugs that May Cause Photosensitivity

Anti-depressants, including Adapin, Asendin, Elavil, Norpramin, Vivactil.

Anti-histamines, including Benadryl.

Anti-microbials, including Bactrim, Fansidar, Septra, the tetracyclines and the doxycyclines.

Anti-parasitics, including Chloroquine and Quinine.

Anti-psychotics, including Haldol, Phenergan, Thorazine.

Diuretics, including Diamox and Lasix.

Hypoglycemics, including Diabinase, Glucotrol, Orinase, Tolinase.

NSAIDs (non-steroidal anti-inflammatory drugs), including Clinoril, Feldene, Naprosyn, Orudis.

WHAT TO DO

Direct ultraviolet light should be avoided when you're taking a drug or using a chemical that makes you photosensitive. If you're having an allergic reaction, try a different brand. If you're unsure, consult your physician.

RESOURCES

"Skin and Sun Savvy," by Paul Gill, Jr., M.D. *Outdoor Life,* May 1989.

The Waterlover's Guide to Marine Medicine, by Paul Gill, Jr., M.D. Simon & Schuster, Rockefeller Center, 1230 Avenue of the Americas, New York, NY 10020.

21 YOUR IMMUNE SYSTEM

"We know that there are immunological effects in humans, though we don't yet know their significance."
— Margaret Kripke, M. D.
Anderson Cancer Center, Houston.

Natural immunity, the ability to fight off disease, can be impaired in some animals who are subjected to excesses of ultraviolet radiation. Do UV rays have that effect on humans? The chances are high that they do.

Specific cells in human skin play a key role in human immunity responses. People with a shortage of these cells are more susceptible to some diseases, including skin cancers. In some people, UVB appears to destroy these protective immune cells. Since UVB causes mutations in normal cells that can lead to cancer, and since UVB might be destroying the immune response that naturally fights cancerous cells, overexposure to sunlight could be a "double negative" in terms of increasing your risk of skin cancer.

WHAT TO DO

Little is known for sure, but much is suspected. Play it safe by reducing your exposure to direct sunlight.

RESOURCE

"Immunogenetic Factors in Skin Cancer," by J. Wayne Streilein. *New England Journal of Medicine,* September 1991.

22 WATER DOESN'T PUT OUT THE FIRE

"Approximately 80% of UV (radiation) penetrates one foot of distilled water, posing the threat of serious sunburn to scuba divers and snorkelers."
— James R. Roberts, M.D.

Swimmers beware. All that water flowing with satisfying coolness over your skin does not protect you from UV radiation. It makes you feel safe, but, in fact, skin that has absorbed a lot of water, from about an hour of swimming, will allow UV rays to penetrate approximately four times better that dry skin. Even water just on the surface of your skin reduces the reflectivity of light and will encourage a sunburn to develop faster and deeper.

Humidity, too, plays a role in sunburn. You'll burn faster on a hot, humid day than on a hot, dry day.

WHAT TO DO

Use a water-proof sunscreen when swimming or when exposing your skin to sunlight on a high humidity day. Use a sunscreen with a high SPF, and reapply it often—at least every two hours.

RESOURCE

Management of Wilderness and Environmental Emergencies, edited by Paul Auerbach, M.D. and Edward Geehr, M.D. The C.V. Mosby Company, 11830 Westline Industrial Drive, St. Louis, MO 63146.

23 TAN, DON'T BURN

"All tanning is visible evidence of toxic injury."

– National Institutes of Health,
convened panel of dermatologists

Genetically, you were programmed with a fixed number of melanocytes, the pigment-producing cells in your epidermis. Dark-skinned people have lots of melanocytes while light-skinned people have few. Your number of melanocytes determines your ability to tan. The dark pigment produced by melanocytes, called melanin, causes tanning and blocks the transmission of UVB into the deeper layers of your skin.

Tanning is a two phase phenomenon. The first phase is stimulated by UVA, involves immediate darkening of existing melanin, and lasts only a few hours. It often goes unnoticed. The second phase, stimulated by UVB, involves a lasting increase in the amount of melanin. This is a true tan. UVA, over a long period of time, will also produce a similar tan. Without repeated exposure to UV rays, tans fade over several weeks due to the constant natural loss and replacement of epidermal cells.

Tanned skin burns less easily than non-tanned skin. Quantitatively, tans provide an SPF of 2 to 4. Otherwise there are no known health benefits to tanning. And almost everyone requires at least a modest sunburn in order to initiate tanning. People who tan poorly, or not at all, are at the greatest risk for developing skin cancer or other degenerative skin disorders while attempting to acquire a tan.

RESOURCES

Management of Wilderness and Environmental Emergencies, edited by Paul Auerbach, M.D., and Edward Geehr, M.D. The C. V. Mosby Company, 11830 Westline Industrial Drive, St. Louis, MO 63146.

The Waterlover's Guide to Marine Medicine, by Paul Gill, Jr., M.D. Simon & Schuster, Rockefeller Center, 1230 Avenue of the Americas, New York NY 10020.

24 UNDERSTAND SPF

SPF, Sun Protection Factor, tells you how long you can stay exposed to sunlight before you burn, compared to exposure time without a sunscreen. For example, if you would burn in 10 minutes, an SPF of 10 allows you, theoretically, to stay in sunlight 10 x 10, or 100 minutes, before burning occurs. The number varies directly with the concentration of the ingredients used in the sunscreen, but SPFs are an average and not an exact number. In actual use, you need to consider an SPF to be only 50% to 75% as effective as the number indicates. For example, a sunscreen with SPF 15 should be considered, to be safe, to give you 8 times more safe exposure, instead of 15 times.

Although it seems that an SPF of 15 would do for almost anyone, studies show that higher SPFs offer greater protection, especially during the first few hours of exposure to UV radiation.

SPF measures UVB protection, not UVA. No rating system approved by the FDA tells you how well you are protected against UVA. A system for rating UVA protection, based on the time it takes for a phototoxic reaction to occur on photosensitized skin, is being considered. If approved, UVA protection will be rated as a PPF number (phototoxic protection factor).

WHAT TO DO

1. Most adults should choose an SPF of at least 15 if they want to tan, and SPF 25 if they want to prevent tanning.

2. If you're fair-skinned or anticipate exposure for an extended period of time, always choose an SPF higher than 15.

3. Because childhood sunburns increase the risk of skin cancer later in life, children should use an SPF of at least 25 starting at six months of age. (Keep children less than six months of age out of direct sunlight.)

4. If a PPF rating is approved, choose the highest PPF you can find.

RESOURCES

Bill Shields, chemist, developer of Ultra One sunscreen for Sawyer Products. Call (800) 356-7811 for more information.

The Medical Letter on Drugs and Therapeutics, edited by Mark Abramowicz, M.D. Volume 35, 11 June 1993. 1000 Main Street, New Rochelle, NY 10801.

University of California, Berkeley Wellness Letter, June 1993. Sub info: P. O. Box 420148, Palm Beach, FL 32142. (904) 445-6414.

25 USE A SUNSCREEN

Sunscreens contain compounds that absorb UV rays before they harm you. The best products have two or more active ingredients that work against UVA and UVB radiation. Para-aminobenzoic acid (PABA) and its derivatives (padimate A and padimate O) are the most common sunscreen ingredients, but they cause skin irritations in many people and have little benefit against UVA. Non-PABA products which contain benzophenones (oxybenzone), cinnamates (octyl methoxycinnamate), salicylates, or anthraniline are very effective sunscreens. The benzophenones are especially effective against UVA. (Read the label on your sunscreen.)

Sunscreens are formulated with bases of lotion, cream, gel, oil or wax. There is no UV protective benefit to a specific base. The choice is personal, usually determined by which one feels best to you. Some bases, however, move around on your skin or off your skin more quickly via heat, sweat and water. Some experts refer to the movement of sunscreen bases as the "migratory factor."

Some sunscreens, depending on the base, are labeled "water-resistant" or "water-proof." Water-resistance implies the product will work for approximately 45 minutes of swimming or heavy sweating. Water-proof sunscreens should be working after 80 minutes under the same conditions.

In 1989, the sunscreen Photoflex (from Allergan Herbert) became the first "broad spectrum" product (protective against UVA and UVB) to become available in the United States. The sunscreens Shade UVAGuard (from Schering-Plough) and Ultra One (from Sawyer) now also offer maximum broad spectrum protection. Ultra One offers an additional benefit of maximum drying on your skin instead of absorption, which provides longer lasting protection.

WHAT TO DO

1. Choose a sunscreen that protects maximally against UVA and UVB radiation.

2. Choose a sunscreen with a base that resists "migration."

3. Before coating your body with a sunscreen, apply it to a small area, about the size of your hand, and wait an hour to see if you develop a rash or other skin irritation that indicates you're allergic to that particular screen. If you are allergic, try a different brand.

4. If you're swimming or sweating a lot, use a water-resistant or water-proof sunscreen.

5. If you're taking a medication, check with your doctor or pharmacist concerning possible side-effects with sunscreens or sunlight.

RESOURCES

Kurt Avery, Sawyer Products, P. O. Box 188, Safety Harbor, FL 34695.

Management of Wilderness and Environmental Emergencies, edited by Paul Auerbach, M.D., and Edward Geehr, M.D., The C. V. Mosby Company, 11830 Westline Industrial Drive, St. Louis, MO 63146.

26 APPLY SUNSCREENS CORRECTLY

"The only two realistic solutions to prevention of overexposure to solar radiation are limitation of exposure time and use of effective sunscreens."
— James R. Roberts, M.D., University of Cincinnati Hospital.

The SPF is based on a uniform sunscreen covering of your skin of approximately 2mg/square centimeter. If you aren't uniformly coated, you aren't uniformly protected. The average adult wearing an average swimsuit should use an average of one ounce (30cc) of screen for one application. Proper application is the single most important factor in determining the effectiveness of your sunscreen.

WHAT TO DO

1. For best results, apply sunscreen when your skin is dry. Moisture mixes with the screen and reduces effectiveness.

2. Apply a sunscreen at least 10 minutes, preferably 30-60 minutes, before exposure to sunlight to allow it to dry on your skin.

3. Reapply sunscreens often, at least every two hours, during periods of exposure, especially between the hours of 10A.M. and 3P.M.

4. Don't just smear it on—rub it in.

5. Have someone help you apply screen to hard-to-reach areas such as the middle of your back.

6. Be especially careful to apply a thick coating to areas where skin damage shows up often: nose, tops of ears, behind the ears.

7. Don't forget the part in your hair, and bald spots.

RESOURCES

Bill Shields, chemist, developer of Ultra One sunscreen from Sawyer Products, P. O. Box 188, Safety Harbor, FL 34695. (800) 356-7811 for sunscreen information.

Traveling Healthy, edited by Karl Neumann. 108-48 70th Road, Forest Hills, NY 11375. Volume 2, Number 3.

27 BLOCK THE SUN

Some opaque creams and pastes totally block all UV radiation. In fact, when properly applied, they block all light from reaching your skin. Although some sunscreens with high SPFs are referred to as blocks, only substances that prevent all light from reaching your skin are true sunblocks. Zinc oxide, titanium dioxide, and red veterinary petrolatum are common ingredients in sunblocks. They do not carry an SPF number, and do not irritate skin. Because sunblocks are often messy, greasy, and generally considered unappealing, many people choose not to use them. Some products, however, are offered in designer colors to match the frames of your sunglasses or your swimsuit.

Other substances can be used as sunblocks if commercially manufactured products are unavailable: ashes from a fire, charcoal, mud or clay mixed into a paste, axle grease. Your "unappeal factor" will go way up.

WHAT TO DO

1. Apply sunblocks thickly, so that none of your skin shows through, similar to the way a clown applies make-up.

2. Apply sunblocks on your nose, lips, the tops of your ears, or other sensitive areas, where exposure tends to be highest.

3. Use a sunblock if you are especially sensitive to sunscreens.

RESOURCES

Sunblock creams available commercially include the trade names: A-Fil, Covermark, Clinique, Reflecta, RV Paque, and Shadow.

28 DON'T GIVE THE SUN ANY LIP

Human lips are a favorite place for skin damage to appear later in life. Lips are a favorite place for you to forget to apply sunscreen, or to apply sunscreen too thin because it doesn't taste very good. Even when applied appropriately, sunscreen comes off your lips faster than any other body part due to lip-licking, lip-wiping, eating and drinking.

WHAT TO DO

Watch for a freckly, scaly, pinkish growth on your lips. If it goes away in a week or so, you're OK. If it becomes sore or painful, refuses to heal, changes color, or grows in size, check in with your doctor.

Buy a lip balm/sunscreen with an SPF of 25, and use it often while your lips are exposed to UV radiation. The taste of many lip balms is OK, or at least acceptable. Make sure your lip balm has an SPF rating—many don't.

RESOURCE

Cancer Information Clearinghouse, Building 31, Room 10A18, 9000 Rockville Pike, Bethesda, MD 20205. (800) 4-CANCER.

29 DRESS FOR THE SUN

You can wear clothing from head to toe and still sunburn.

Wear clothing that has a tight weave. Hold your clothing up to a bright light. The more light showing through, the more ultraviolet radiation is getting through. Tightly woven cotton tends to offer more protection than tightly woven polyesters. A pair of blue denim jeans can provide an SPF of over 1000. A loosely woven nylon shirt can provide an SPF as little as 4 or 5.

Wear clothing that fits loosely. When clothing is stretched over part of your body, the UV protection is reduced, sometimes dramatically. One garment, say a shirt, can be three or four times more protective at your waist than it is where it stretches over your shoulder.

Wear dark clothing. Dyed fabric, in general, blocks more UV light than undyed fabric. A dark garment can provide up to twice the protection of a lighter color.

Keep your clothing dry. No matter the weave or color or material, water (including sweat) enhances the transparency of any garment. A T-shirt can offer an SPF between 7 and 20 when dry, but only 5 to 10 when wet.

RESOURCE

Robert Sayre, PhD, biophysicist, University of Tennessee Center for the Health Sciences, Memphis.

30 SPECIAL CLOTHING

Even though long-sleeved shirts and long pants offer more protection than shorts and T-shirts, you may not be comfortable on a warm sunny day in the protective clothing you own, and you may not be getting the amount of protection you want. Some emerging manufacturers specialize in clothing that is loose and comfortable with the fibers and the weaving method both chosen for maximum UV protection.

Frogwear of Tempe, AZ, offers shirts, pants, shorts, jackets and hats (adult and children sizes) made with fibers treated for enhanced moisture evaporation to keep you cooler on hot days. With claims to block out 98.5% of all UVB and 97% of all UVA, Frogwear has been endorsed by The American Melanoma Foundation.

Sun Precautions of Seattle, WA, offers a full range of clothing (adult and children sizes), including hooded jackets and gloves, made with specially treated fibers that block over

97% of all harmful UV radiation. In addition, they offer sun accessories, including sunscreens and sunglasses.

With special UV protective clothing, you may find yourself spending more money than you intended to, but you'll find yourself comfortable and well-protected from UV radiation.

RESOURCES

Frogskin, Inc., P. O. Box 25364, Tempe, AZ 85285-5364. (800) 354-0203.

Sun Precautions, Inc., 105 2nd Avenue North, Seattle, WA 98109. (800) 882-7860.

31 HAT TIPS

"Anything shorter than three inches isn't very effective."
– Madhu Pathak, PhD, dermatologist
Harvard Medical School.

Three inches of brim on your hat, all the way around, is required to provide enough shade to prevent skin damage. That's because baseball caps, even caps with extra long front brims, protect your face but still allow the sun to reach your ears and neck. Basal cell carcinoma appear most often on the face, ears and neck. Up to 85% of direct UV light can be blocked with a wide brim. For some reason, probably due to greater light dispersion, floppy brims offer a little more protection that rigid brims.

An option is a commercially-made front-brimmed cap with a French Foreign Legion-type flap sewn on the back to protect your neck and ears (from Frogskin, Inc. and Solar Protective Factory, Inc. and Sun Precautions, Inc.). You can make your own, or you can make do in a pinch by placing a bandanna or other piece of cloth under your baseball cap with most of the cloth hanging down over your neck and ears.

Traveler's Checklist of Sharon, CT, offers cotton hats that fold up small and pop open to form a protective hat with 5 inch brim. Two hats come packaged with a UV Sensometer (see 41. UV Sensometer) as The Safe Sun Kit.

RESOURCES

Frogskin, Inc., P. O. Box 25364, Tempe, AZ 85285-5364. (800) 354-0203.

Sun Precautions, Inc. 105 2nd Avenue North, Seattle, WA 98109. (800) 882-7860.

Sun Protective Factory, Inc., 564 LaSierra Drive, Suite 18, Sacramento, CA 95864. (800) 786-2562.

Traveler's Checklist, 335 Cornwall Bridge Road, Sharon, CT 06069. (203) 364-0144.

UV AND YOUR EYES

32 SOLAR RETINITIS

"Since the time of Plato, visual disturbances have been associated with sun viewing."

–Yannuzzi, et al.

Your retina, the innermost part of your eye, the part that receives images directly from the lens of your eye, is your immediate instrument of vision. Any inflamed condition of the retina is called retinitis. Although solar retinitis most often results in people who have stared too long at an eclipse of the sun, an increasing number of cases are being reported in patients who have been merely sunbathing or exercising in direct sunlight during periods of reduced ozone concentration. What happens is this: your eye's lens, working much like a magnifying glass, focuses solar radiation on your retina, and burns it.

Those people affected usually have normal vision or better than normal vision, but, soon after exposure to the sun, signs of eye damage develop that include: reduced ability to see, a blind spot in the field of vision, an intolerance for bright light, and seeing unusual colors or shapes.

WHAT TO DO

Some people who develop solar retinitis never fully recover, but most sufferers regain normal eyesight within 3-9 months. All patients so far have had one common predisposing factor: they were not wearing sunglasses.

RESOURCE

Solar Retinopathy, by Lawrence Yannuzzi, M.D., Yale Fisher, M.D., Jason Slakter, M.D., and Arlin Krueger, PhD. A thesis presented at the American Ophthalmological Society.

33 CATARACTS

"More than a million cataract operations are performed each year in the U.S., accounting for about 12% of the entire Medicare budget."
—From the editors of the *University of California Berkeley Wellness Letter*

Cataracts are cloudings of the lens of the human eye, or the capsule of the lens, or both. As cataracts develop, your ability to see diminishes, and finally goes away. Surgery can often restore sight, with the use of eyeglasses. Not long ago, cataracts were considered an unavoidable result of aging, but it is now believed they can be postponed, even prevented. The three main contributors to cataracts, other than aging, are 1) cigarette smoking, 2) a diet poor in vitamins C and E, beta carotene, and other antioxidants . . . and 3) lifelong exposure to ultraviolet light.

Dark-skinned people are less likely to develop skin cancer, but dark-eyed people are more likely to develop cataracts, from UV rays, than blue, green and gray-eyed people. The reason probably lies in the fact that dark eyes have more melanin, and melanin absorbs more solar radiation, and, over time, more damage is done to the lens of the eye.

WHAT TO DO

The darker your eyes, the more important your choice of sunglasses. Sunglasses should protect your eyes from all UV rays, at least 75% of visible light, and from violet/blue light, too (which may further degenerate the retina). Wide brimmed hats add further protection for your eyes.

RESOURCES

Traveling Healthy, Volume 2, Number 3, edited by Karl Neumann, M.D., 108-48 70th Road, Forest Hills, NY 11375.

The Wellness Encyclopedia, by the editors of the *University of California, Berkeley Wellness Letter,* P. O. Box 412, Prince Street Station, New York, NY 10012.

34 SNOWBLINDNESS

Approximately 75% of UVA and UVB is reflected back at you by snow, so your eyes are bombarded with direct UV light and reflected UV light when you're outside on a snow-covered day. UVA can penetrate your eyelids, but it's probably UVB that does most of the damage. Clouds do not protect your eyes. In an hour of high level exposure, or a few hours on bright days, the cornea of your eye can sunburn, and a problem called snowblindness (also called ultraviolet keratitis or photokeratitis) results.

6-12 hours pass before the sensations of snowblindness begin: pain, feeling like sand is in your eyes, sensitivity to light ("blindness"), lots of tears, red eyes, and sometimes eyelid swelling.

Spontaneous healing usually occurs within 24 hours. In the meantime, reducing your pain is the main goal. Flushing eyes gently with cold water and cold compresses on the eyes help. Anti-inflammatory drugs such as aspirin and ibuprofen may help. You may ask your doctor for a topical ophthalmic anesthetic (painkilling eye ointment) or a prescription-strength painkilling drug. Patch the affected eyes to protect them from light. Or you can grin and bear it. If you're not significantly better in 24 hours, see your doctor for sure.

WHAT TO DO

Snowblindness is entirely preventable. Wear sunglasses that protect your eyes from UV light. The sunglasses should wrap-around or, even better, have side shields to protect your eyes from reflected light. Repeated snow-blindness can cause yellowing of the lens of your eye and cataracts.

RESOURCE

Management of Wilderness and Environmental Emergencies, edited by Paul Auerbach, M.D.., and Edward Geehr, M.D. The C. V. Mosby Company, 11830 Westline Industrial Drive, St. Louis, MO 63146.

35 WEAR GOOD SUNGLASSES

"A good pair of sunglasses . . . filters out all UVB and at least 99% of UVA."
— Stephen R. Chun, O.D., F.A.A.O.

Ultraviolet light is either filtered out or absorbed by your sunglasses, depending on the lens material, thickness of the lens, and the way the lens is processed. Both plastic and glass lenses can have absorptive tints added for maximum UV protection. For glass, tints are usually added during the early stages of manufacture. Tints are melted into the glass, and they are permanent. For plastic, the tints are added late in the manufacturing process. Tints adhere by surface absorption into the plastic and, being organic compounds, they may fade over time. Tints come in many colors, and range from dark to light. Both plastic and glass can have absorptive coatings added after manufacture. They stick better to glass, but these surface coatings can be scratched off.

How do you know if your sunglasses are good? Unfortunately, it's not as easy as you may think. The darkness of the lens, for instance, is not an indicator of the UV protection. Inadequately treated dark lenses can actually be harmful, offering little protection while keeping your pupils open to long-term damage. Labels on name brands that guarantee protection can usually be trusted. Labels on some imported brands are sometimes worth no more than the paper—or plastic—they're printed on. Your safest bet is to have the effectiveness of your sunglasses checked with a spectrophotometer by your local optometrist or ophthalmologist.

Sunglasses should fit properly, resting on your nose, not on your cheeks. The lens should come as close to your eyes as possible without letting your eyelashes touch the plastic or glass.

In addition, some sunglasses cause image distortion that can lead to eyestrain and headaches. Wraparound lenses are especially susceptible to peripheral distortion. For non-prescription lenses, hold your sunglasses at arm's length and look at a straight line (a doorway, for example). If the straight line is bent through your sunglasses, you are being optically distorted.

RESOURCE

"Wilderness Eye Protection," by Stephen R. Chun, O.D. *Wilderness First Aid,* P. O. Box 1227, Berkeley, CA 94701. Spring 1990 issue.

36 LABELING STANDARDS FOR SUNGLASSES

"The reason for applying tighter UVB limits across the board, even for cosmetic sunglasses, is to make sure the public's health is protected as much as possible."
— Morris Waxler, PhD,
FDA Center for Devices and Radiological Health.

Shopping for a pair of sunglasses that will properly protect your eyes is not easy. Many inexpensive glasses are not labeled or are incorrectly labeled. Even if the label says "Meets ANSI Z80.3 requirements," you are not getting full protection against UVB and UVA. Here's why: The current ANSI standards require only voluntary compliance by sunglass manufacturers—yet they are endorsed by the FDA. Under the present ANSI/FDA system, there are three classes of sunglasses:

• Cosmetic—block at least 70% UVB and 20% UVA.

- General Purpose—block at least 95% UVB and 60% UVA.

- Special Purpose—block at least 99% UVB and 60% UVA.

Based on new evidence of cataracts, solar retinitis and other UV-related eye disorders, Dr. Waxler and other vision researchers believe the present ANSI labeling system to be inadequate. Here's a summary of the newly proposed FDA standard, based on a two-category system:

- Sunglasses—block at least 99% UVB—Adequate to protect the eyes in moderately bright sunlight, such as low-altitude, urban areas in temperate to northern latitudes.

- UV-Blocking Sunglasses—block at least 99% UVB and 99% UVA—Adequate to protect human eyes in bright sunlight such as found in low-elevation snowfields and non-equatorial beaches, if the lenses also block 60 to 90% of visible light. For extremely bright environments such as high-elevation snow or equatorial beaches, the UV-blocking lens should stop 92 to 97 percent of visible light, and have sideshields or goggles. (Glasses with sideshields and goggles should not be used while driving).

Until tighter sunglass standards are in place, only buy "ANSI Special Purpose" sunglasses, and have your existing sunglasses tested for UV blocking effectiveness.

RESOURCES

FDA Consumer, June 1992, p 24.

VisionMonday, May 25, 1992, p 6.

37 TEST YOUR SUNGLASSES

Since UV light is invisible, you cannot tell how effective your sunglasses are by looking at the tint of the lenses. Many sunglasses sold today are not marked for UV protection, and cheap import sunglasses may have inaccurate UV protection labels. Continued use of poor quality sunglasses can do serious damage to your eyes.

If you are using sunglasses purchased several years ago, or are wearing prescription sunglasses, you may have no idea as to how effective they are at screening out the sun's UV rays. However, buying new sunglasses—especially ones with prescription lenses—is expensive, so you don't want to throw away glasses that are working properly.

What To Do

Many optometrists and optical shops now have instruments—UV Photometers—to test the effectiveness of sunglasses. Bring your sunglasses in and have them tested. Usually there is no charge for this service.

If your existing prescription sunglasses are not blocking UV effectively, you can have the lenses treated with a special coating to block nearly 100% of UV. This is a less expensive option than ordering a new set of glasses.

Resource

BPI-Brain Power International produces a "Computer Cal" line of UV Photometers sold to many eye doctors and optical shops. (800) 327-2250.

38 Prescription Sunglasses

If you need prescription lenses to adjust your eyesight, and if you need sunglasses at the same, you've got two choices:

You can get your prescription glasses with photochromic lenses. First introduced by Corning Glass Works in 1964, photochromic lenses have silver and chloride ions included in the glass when its formed. When exposed to ultraviolet or blue light, the ions dissociate and cluster into specks that absorb 100% of the UVB and 93-98% of the UVA radiation. The more light hitting the lens, the darker it grows. Some photochromic lenses are also temperature sensitive, growing darker in cold air and lighter in warm air.

You can get prescription sunglasses, optics with permanent tints, treated for protection against UV rays. Many companies offer a wide variety of prescription sport optics, glasses designed with specific sports in mind (e.g. skiing, biking, fishing).

WHAT TO DO

Some states require all prescription sunglasses to be purchased from a licensed optical dispenser, in which case you have to visit your optician. Some states allow you to place orders directly from manufacturers (see Resources).

RESOURCES

Manufacturers that offer prescription sunglass service include:

Action Optics: (800) 654-6428.

Bausch & Lomb: (800) 828-1930.

Bollé: (800) 554-6686.

Bucci: (800) 999-2822.

Cebe: (800) 543-9124.

Gargoyles: (206) 251-5001.

Hobie: (800) 554-4335.

Julbo: (800) 451-5127.

Revo: (800) 367-7386.

Scott: (800) 292-5874.

Smith: (208) 726-4477.

Sport Visions of Sun Valley: (800) 527-3105.

Vuarnet: (800) 348-0388.

39 OVERGLASSES INSTEAD OF PRESCRIPTION SUNGLASSES

If you wear prescription glasses, you face special problems in protecting your eyes from intense sunlight. With today's higher UV levels you really need eyewear with side protection.

One study reports that up to 40% of UV enters the eye from the sides and tops of conventional prescription sunglasses. Curved "wraparound" style sunglasses are not currently available in prescription form, but one practical alternative is a rectangular wraparound overglass that fits over existing eyeglasses.

A new generation of overglasses are designed to fit comfortably and stylishly over existing eyewear. The sides of these glasses are made of the same polycarbonate material used for the lenses, so peripheral vision is preserved, making them suitable for driving. The glasses come in a variety of tints and frame colors. Some models offer polarized lenses, while others block blue-violet light as well as UVB and UVA.

RESOURCES

For information on wraparound sunglasses that fit over existing eyewear, contact these companies:

EYE Communications, 1241 West 9th Street, Upland, CA 91786. (800) 247-5731.

Rocky Mountain High Sports Glasses, 8121 N. Central Park, Skokie, IL 60076. (708) 679-1012.

Vision Products, 1301 Willow Way, Garland, TX 75043. (800) 332-2106.

40 SAVING FACE WITH EYEWEAR

Some eyewear products offer unique UV protection features. Here are some examples:

For mountaineering or skiing in very bright, high-altitude snow conditions, consider using a product with a built-in nose protector. Recreational Equipment, Inc. (REI) sells a product they call "Glacier Overglasses" that have a removable nose protector flap to shade your nose. These overglasses may be worn over your regular glasses. Another handy product from REI for bright environments is a set of "Clip-on Side Protectors" that will add sideshielding to any set of ordinary sunglasses.

For something a bit more "eye-catching" you may want to buy a pair of Platipus sport goggles from Eye Communications. These goggles are actually a wrap-around style of sunglasses that include a visor-style sun shield attached to the top of the goggles. It's like having a sun visor built into your sunglasses. The stiff plastic visors come in a variety of colors, providing your nose and face with protective shade.

RESOURCES

Glacier Overglasses (stock #409-131, $17.00) and Clip-On Side Protectors (stock #409-032, $2.95) available from REI: (800) 426-4840.

Platipus Sport Goggles, available from Eye Communications: (800) 247-5731.

UV AND YOUR LIFESTYLE

41 UV SENSOMETERS

Ultraviolet light is invisible to the human eye. Normally you don't see or feel the effects of UV overexposure until it is too late—then you've got a sunburn or sore eyes from UV damage.

One way to visualize the relative intensity of UV levels is to use a low-cost, re-usable UV monitor, called the UV Sensometer. This gadget looks like a plastic credit card, but, instead of a magnetic strip, it has a strip with a UV-sensitive chemical that changes color. You simply hold the card up to the sun for ten seconds and the white strip changes color to indicate the UV intensity—darker shades of purple indicate stronger UV levels. (To make another reading, you will need to cover the card or keep it indoors for several minutes to let it turn white again.) While the Sensometer gives only relative readings, it is still useful for testing the effectiveness of your sunglasses and your sunscreen lotion. If you put the card behind the lenses of your sunglasses, it should remain white if the glasses block 100 percent of the UV rays. Smearing lotion over the strip will give you an idea how effective your sunscreen is, too. Another good experiment is to compare the intensity of UV rays at mid-day with levels later in the evening. You can also use the device to convince your-self that UV is still present on cloudy days.

RESOURCES

The UV Sensometer is priced at $4.95. It is available from two companies:

Eye Communications, 1241 West 9th Street, Upland, CA 91786. (800) 247-5731 or (714) 949-1494.

Optiwear, P.O. Box 132, Syracuse, NY 13206. (315) 463-0055.

42 BABIES AND BRIGHT SUNLIGHT DON'T MIX

The delicate skin of babies and young children is especially sensitive to the intense sun. A single bad sunburn during childhood can double your child's risk of skin cancer later in life. Babies under one year of age should not be exposed to direct sunlight. Protect them by using a covered stroller, and be sure to keep them in shade at picnics and other outdoor gatherings.

The strong chemicals in some sunscreens can also irritate a newborn's skin. For this reason, many experts do not recommend applying sunscreens to babies less than six months old. When you start using a sunscreen on an infant, you may want to choose one that contains inert zinc oxide instead of the stronger chemicals. Many companies now make sunscreens just for babies and young children.

Babies and young children are less aware of protecting their eyes than adults, and are more susceptible to irreversible solar eye damage. Several manufacturers make sunglasses especially for infants and young children.

WHAT TO DO

1. Keep babies under one year out of direct sunlight.

2. Never use baby oil as a sunscreen, and don't use sunscreens at all on babies under six months of age.

3. Try to keep toddlers out of the sun from 10 A.M. to 3 P.M.

4. Create shade for your baby—take advantage of covered patios, umbrellas, and shade trees.

5. Buy your children their own sunglasses, and wear yours as an example.

RESOURCES

Sunscreen: Summer Stuff from Sawyer Products, P. O. Box 188, Safety Harbor, FL 34695.

Sunglasses: Baby Optics (800) 962-6874. Scott (800) 292-5874. Solar Sense (800) 285-0785. Vuarnet (800) 348-0388.

43 TEACH YOUR CHILDREN WELL

"The regular use of appropriate sunscreens during the first 18 years of life would reduce a child's lifetime risk of developing sun related skin cancers by 78%."

– Robert Stern, M.D., Harvard University

Forget what your parents told you—children don't need direct sunlight to grow normally, sunlight has little to do with good health in children, sunlight does not help you develop a pretty complexion. Children are not little adults. Direct sunlight is even worse for children than it is for grown-ups. Kids burn faster, and cumulative skin damage starts with the first exposure.

According to the Skin Cancer Foundation, 80% of your lifetime exposure to skin-damaging ultraviolet light occurs during the first 18-20 years of life. Intense one-day exposure during a child's lifetime, say a day at the beach unprotected, may be more harmful than numerous short-term exposures. But the damage may not show up for 30 years.

TEACH YOUR CHILDREN TO:

1. . . use sunscreen, just like you teach them to brush their teeth. For young children, screens with a milky lotion or cream base feel better to their skin, do not contain alcohol which can sting, and it's easier to see where it has been applied compared to clear lotions. Sawyer

Products offers Summer Stuff, a PABA and fragrance free sunscreen for kids, SPF 25, with UVA and UVB protection. The screen comes in Pink Pizazz, Blue Blast, Green Slime and Wacky White, colors that fade fast and harmlessly on skin. Each bottle comes with a sticky label you can write your child's name on to personalize their bottle. Each package contains a crayon and sun-related educational coloring book.

2. . . apply sunscreen carefully, covering all exposed skin, especially their nose, ears, lips and neck, but avoiding the upper and lower eyelids. Kids tend to rub screen into their eyes. Not all screens are eye-irritating, but many are.

3. . . wear sunglasses. Eyelids are the thinnest and most delicate part of the body. UV damage to eyes can start with a child's first exposure.

RESOURCES

Sawyer Products, P. O. Box 188, Safety Harbor, FL 34695.

Traveling Healthy, edited by Karl Neumann, M.D. 108-48 70th Road, Forest Hills, NY 11375. Volume 2, Number 3.

44 UV AND YOUR VACATION

Vacations! Time to break away for some rest, relaxation, and recreation. Time for some fresh air and sunshine—but not too much sunshine!

Before booking that plane ticket, consider how the choice of date and location affects your UVB exposure. You can reduce your sunburn and cancer risks by picking your vacation time or vacation spot. Here are some examples, using UV Index values calculated from the UV B-WARE™ computer program:

Let's say you're thinking about some beach time in Acapulco. Your first inclination is to go around spring break, on March 20. A computerized estimate of UV levels for Acapulco at that time shows a UV Index of 10.2, near the top of the scale. However if you visit Acapulco around January 20, only two months earlier, the UV Index should be only 7.2—a full 30% lower.

Suppose you are a skier considering a spring skiing vacation during the first week in April. A quick check of estimated UVB levels with the computer gives these Index readings:

Aspen, Colorado	5.9
Salt Lake City, Utah	5.6
Jackson Hole, Wyoming	4.8
Banff, Alberta	3.5

Skiing in Wyoming could cut your UV dose 19% compared to Colorado, while a trip to the Canadian Rockies would reduce levels by 31%.

RESOURCE

The UV B-WARE™ program for PC compatibles costs $39.95. It is available from Save the Planet Software, P.O. Box 45, Pitkin, CO 81241. (303) 641-5035.

45 CREATE MORE SHADE IN YOUR BACKYARD

As ozone levels drop, you may want to develop more shady areas for your own yard. This way you and your family can still enjoy being outside, while being protected from excessive UV rays. Adding shade can be accomplished by landscaping (planting more trees) and by "home improvement" projects that involve the construction of covers or canopies over decks and patio areas.

When planning these projects, keep in mind the angle and path of both the summer sun and winter sun. What you want are trees and structures that deliver maximum shade during the summer months, but are designed and placed in such a way as to provide warm and mild sunlight during the winter. Planting deciduous trees on the south side of your house is one way to do this. During summer they will give you welcome shade when you need it, and in the fall, they'll drop their leaves, permitting the winter sun to brighten your windows and help lower your heating bill.

Deck and patio areas should be covered with high roofs open on the sides for summer ventilation. Deck and patio floors should be stained or painted a dark color or constructed of non-reflective material. Screens that keep out bugs help keep out some UV radiation.

RESOURCE

The Sunset Publishing Company produces a fine series of home and garden improvement books that are filled with ideas, photos, and plans for patio roofs, decks, fences, and garden projects. Available at most bookstores, or contact: Sunset Publishing, 80 Willow Road, Menlo Park CA 94025. (415) 321-3600.

46 PARASOLS: SHADE YOU CAN CARRY

Sun umbrellas—parasols—are not a new idea. The word "parasol" comes from the French language and means "to ward off the sun." Using a sun umbrella is good idea, whether you are hiking in the desert or hanging around the beach. While you can use an ordinary umbrella to provide modest protection, the ideal parasol should be made out of a fabric that effectively stops UV rays. The "UV Block Umbrella" is manufactured by the Solar Protective Factory, Inc. This sun umbrella uses the company's proprietary sun-blocking fabric: Solarweave. Solarweave stops 99% of UVB and 60% of UVA, and retains its UV opacity even after washing or use as a rain umbrella. The "Parasol" is made from Solumbra, a fabric developed by Sun Precautions, Inc., that blocks over 97%

of UVA and UVB rays. Solumbra's UV-blocking ability is not destroyed by rain or washing.

Remember: parasols and beach umbrellas do not prevent skin damage from reflected UV radiation. You should still be wearing a sunscreen on exposed skin.

RESOURCES

The Parasol is available from: Sun Precautions, Inc., 105 2nd Avenue North, Seattle, WA 98109. (800) 882-7860.

The UV Block Umbrella is available from: Solar Protective Factory, Inc., 564 LaSierra Drive, Suite 18, Sacramento, CA 95864. (800) 786-2562.

47 BOOT THE BOOTH

"Contrary to popular belief, tanning salons are not a safe alternative to sun exposure."

— Mayo Clinic Health Letter

According to manufacturers of tanning booths and sunlamps, and operators of tanning salons, you can get an artificially-induced tan from light sources that emit mainly UVA radiation, which is true. And artificially-induced tans from booths are indistinguishable from sun-induced tans. However, you should have concerns about tanning salons: 1) There are no controls to guarantee the light sources are what they're claimed to be, and 2) UVA rays, which penetrate deeper into your skin than UVB, are now known to be unsafe. UVA prematurely ages skin, probably promotes cataracts, induces phototoxic reactions more often that UVB, and augments the cancer-causing effects of UVB. For those reasons, the American Academy of Dermatology discourages the use of artificial UV sources for cosmetic purposes.

The Federal Drug Administration (FDA) estimates that a half hour under a sunlamp can be as detrimental as a half hour on the streets of Washington, DC, at high noon.

RESOURCES

Management of Wilderness and Environmental Emergencies, edited by Paul Auerbach, MD, and Edward Geehr, MD.

"Sun Struck," by Mary Roach. Health, May/June 1992.

48 EAT ENOUGH VITAMIN C, E AND BETA-CAROTENE

"No firm answer can yet be given."
> – University of California,
> Berkeley Wellness Letter, May, 1990.

Free radicals are unstable molecules created by your body by several normal chemical processes. Creation of free radicals gets a boost by some environmental influences including cigarette smoke and solar radiation. Being "incomplete" chemically, free radicals take pieces of other molecules, which causes the production of abnormal compounds that probably play a role in the development of cancer and other diseases.

Vitamins C and E, and beta-carotene (a member of a large group of nutrients called carotenoids) are antioxidants. Antioxidants are substances with the unique property of being willing and able to destroy free radicals. Do they help prevent cancer? Nobody knows for sure, but everyone agrees your body needs an adequate supply of all nutrients to stay healthy.

How much do you need? The National Research Council determines the Recommended Daily Allowance (RDA) of nutrients. The RDA for vitamin C is 60mg. Eating more vitamin C than you need is relatively harmless since the vitamin is water-soluble and your body excretes what it can't use. For vitamin E the RDA is 8-10mg. Vitamin E is fat-soluble, your body stores it, and too much can become toxic. Nobody knows exactly where vitamin E toxicity begins. There is no RDA for beta-carotene.

Your best bet is to eat plenty of healthy food. Consume at least five servings of fruit and vegetables every day. Antioxidant-rich foods are typically colorful: orange, yellow and dark green.

RESOURCES

University of California, Berkeley Wellness Letter, P. O. Box 420148, Palm Coast, FL 32142. Volume 6, Issue 5.

Eating For Endurance, by Ellen Coleman, Bull Publishing Company, P. O. Box 208, Palo Alto, CA 94302.

49 DON'T BUY OZONE-EATING CHEMICAL PRODUCTS

Many ozone-destroying products are still on store shelves today. While politicians and chemical executives squabble over phaseout timetables, you can vote with your pocketbook today. For your safety and the safety of future generations, please do not buy products that contain CFCs, HCFCs, halons, carbon tetrachloride, methyl bromide, or methyl chloroform (sometimes called 1,1,1 trichloroethylene). Read the labels on chemical containers before you buy. Also avoid dry cleaning establishments that have not yet stopped using carbon tetrachloride and methyl chloroform.

WHAT TO DO

Here is a partial checklist of products to avoid:

1. Halon fire extinguishers.

2. New cars that still use R-12 Freon in the air conditioner.

3. Do-it-yourself pressure cans of R-12 to put in car air conditioners.

4. Boat horns, VCR-head cleaners, electronic cleaning sprays that contain CFCs.

5. Rigid plastic foam products: Cups, plates, building insulation, etc.

6. Many household products that still contain ozone-eating chemicals—fabric protectors, stain removers, solvents, and many pesticides.

7. Electronic products made in China—Although U.S., Canadian, Japanese, and European electronics manufacturers have quit using CFCs to clean microchips and circuit boards, Chinese manufacturers continue to use these harmful chemicals.

50 HELP RECLAIM CFCs IN EXISTING PRODUCTS

Chemical manufacturers are starting to reduce the production of CFCs and other ozone-destroying chemicals, as a result of new laws and the adoption of substitute chemicals. You can help by making sure that the CFCs in existing products are returned for proper CFC reclamation.

WHAT TO DO

1. Be sure your car's air conditioner is serviced at a repair shop that uses equipment to remove CFCs, and returns these CFCs for safe disposal or recycling. Don't junk an old car without first removing the Freon from the air conditioner.

2. Take similar actions when servicing or disposing of refrigerators and air conditioner units. Under the new Clean Air Act, it is no longer legal to simply dump an old air conditioner, freezer, or refrigerator. Call your city or county government, or check with the Environmental Protection Agency (EPA) Hotline. U.S. EPA Stratospheric Ozone Information Hotline: (800) 296-1996.

3. Don't throw your halon fire extinguishers in the trash. Keep them until the EPA has implemented a halon recapture program. To find out when such a program will be available, call the Halon Recycling Corporation at (800) 258-1283.

Thank you !

THE 10 UV PROTECTION ESSENTIALS

DON'T LEAVE HOME WITHOUT THEM

Our sun shines down as a source of joy, life and power. You want to enjoy and utilize the sun's power, but keep in mind it can be destructive. Save your skin and protect your eyes. Know and protect your solar environment. Keep the UV protection basics in mind:

1. Adequate Hat

2. Proper Clothing

3. Good Sunglasses or Overglasses

4. Effective Sunscreen or Sunblock

5. Protective Lip Balm

6. Awareness of Your Solar Environment

7. Awareness of UV Health Hazards

8. A Healthy Diet

9. Knowledge of Ozone-Saving Actions

10. A Decision to Live Well

INDEX